THE REVERSAL DIABETES COOKBOOK

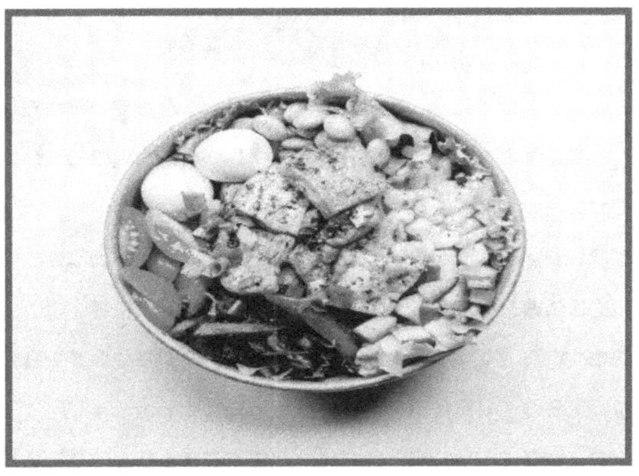

Culinary Adventure on Blood Sugar Control

Jasmine Kurt

TABLE OF CONTENTS

TABLE OF CONTENTS

How to Use this Cookbook

Here's a simple guide to using this diabetes reversal cookbook effectively in five easy steps:

Familiarise Yourself with this Cookbook:
Start by reading the introduction and any explanatory sections provided by this cookbook author. Understand the goals of this cookbook, its approach to managing diabetes, and the types of recipes it offers.
Review the Recipe Categories:
Explore the different sections of this cookbook to see the variety of recipes available. Categories may include breakfast, lunch, dinner, snacks, desserts, and more. Take note of recipes that appeal to you and fit your dietary preferences and restrictions.
Select Recipes Based on Dietary Goals:
When choosing recipes, take your preferences and nutritional objectives into account. Look for recipes that focus on whole, nutrient-dense ingredients, and are lower in refined sugars and carbohydrates. Pay attention to portion sizes and meal balance to help regulate blood sugar levels.
Gather Ingredients and Follow Instructions:
Once you've chosen a recipe, carefully read through the ingredient list and instructions. Make a list of any ingredients you need to purchase and gather them before starting to cook. Follow the recipe instructions step by step, ensuring accuracy in measurements and cooking techniques.
Enjoy and Evaluate:

Once you've prepared the recipe, take time to enjoy the meal. Pay attention to flavours, textures, and overall satisfaction. After trying the recipe, evaluate its suitability for your tastes and dietary needs. Keep notes on recipes you particularly enjoy and those you may want to modify in the future.

By following these steps, you can effectively utilise this diabetes reversal cookbook to explore new recipes, incorporate healthier eating habits, and support your journey towards managing diabetes effectively through diet and lifestyle changes.

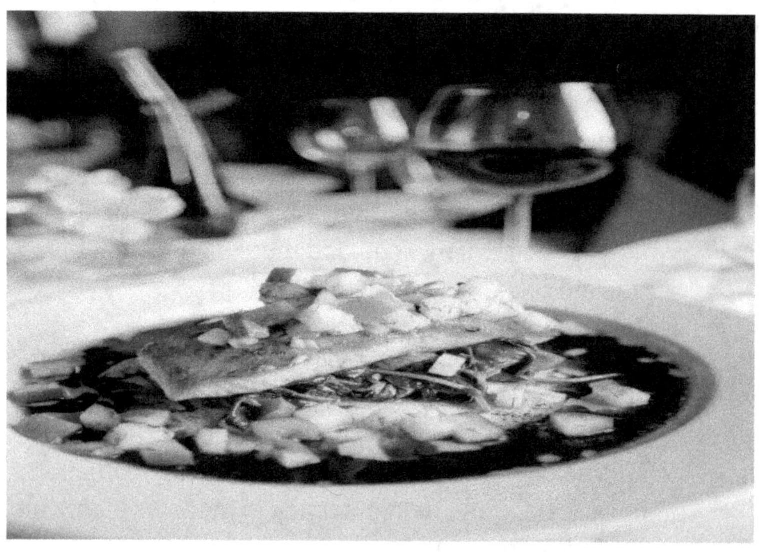

INTRODUCTION

Welcome to a culinary journey that transcends the boundaries of traditional cookbooks – the "Reversal Diabetes Cookbook." This exceptional guide is not just a compilation of recipes but a groundbreaking approach to transforming the way we perceive and interact with food in the context of diabetes management and potential reversal.

Crafted with precision and a profound understanding of nutritional science, this cookbook is more than a collection of delectable dishes. It's a manifesto of empowerment for individuals determined to reclaim control over their health and reverse the course of diabetes through the medium of a well-curated, diverse, and utterly delicious culinary experience.

In the pages that follow, you'll discover a symphony of flavours meticulously orchestrated to not only tantalise your taste buds but to strategically support metabolic health. Each recipe is a testament to the idea that managing diabetes doesn't mean compromising on the joys of eating; instead, it's an opportunity to explore a world of vibrant, nutrient-rich ingredients that can play a pivotal role in transforming your well-being.

The "Reversal Diabetes Cookbook" transcends the conventional boundaries of dietary restrictions, offering a harmonious fusion of innovation and tradition. It's an invitation to embrace the profound impact that mindful eating can have on blood sugar levels and overall health. Whether you're embarking on a journey to reverse Type 2 diabetes or seeking optimal management strategies for Type 1, this cookbook is your compass, guiding you through a culinary landscape where health and flavour coexist seamlessly.

Get ready to embark on a gastronomic adventure that not only nourishes your body but also reshapes your relationship with food. The "Reversal Diabetes Cookbook" is not just a recipe collection; it's a transformative companion on your path to wellness, promising a vibrant and flavorful way forward in the pursuit of reversing diabetes.

CHAPTER ONE

Understanding Diabetes

What is diabetes

Diabetes is a chronic medical condition characterised by elevated blood sugar levels due to the body's inability to produce or effectively use insulin. Insulin, produced by the pancreas, helps regulate blood sugar by allowing cells to absorb glucose for energy. There are two main types of diabetes: Type 1 and Type 2.

Type 1 Diabetes:

Cause: Thought to be an autoimmune response where the body attacks and destroys insulin-producing beta cells in the pancreas.

Onset: Typically diagnosed in childhood or adolescence.

Treatment: Needs constant insulin administration via needles or an insulin pump.

Type 2 Diabetes:

Cause: Linked to genetic factors, lifestyle choices, and obesity. The body becomes insulin resistant, and the pancreas may not produce enough insulin.

Onset: Often develops in adulthood, but increasingly diagnosed in younger individuals.

Treatment: Lifestyle modifications like diet and exercise, oral medications, and sometimes insulin.

Common Symptoms of Diabetes:

Increased thirst and hunger

Frequent urination

Unexplained weight loss

Fatigue

Blurred vision

Complications of Diabetes:

Cardiovascular Issues: Diabetes can contribute to heart disease, stroke, and high blood pressure.

Nerve Damage (Neuropathy): Diabetes can cause tingling or numbness in extremities.

Kidney Damage (Nephropathy): Diabetes is a leading cause of kidney failure.

Eye Problems (Retinopathy): High blood sugar can damage the blood vessels in the retina, leading to vision problems.

Prevention and Management:

Healthy Lifestyle: Regular exercise, a balanced diet, and weight management play crucial roles.

Medication: Insulin, oral medications, and other drugs may be prescribed based on the type and severity of diabetes.

Monitoring Blood Sugar: Regular blood sugar monitoring is essential for managing diabetes effectively.

Education and Support: Understanding the condition, its management, and seeking support from healthcare professionals are vital.

Challenges:

Adherence to treatment plans

Continuous blood sugar monitoring

Lifestyle changes

In conclusion, understanding diabetes involves recognizing its types, symptoms, and complications. Management requires a holistic approach, incorporating lifestyle changes, medication, and regular monitoring, emphasising the importance of patient education and support in achieving optimal outcomes. Regular medical check-ups are crucial for early detection and intervention.

CHAPTER TWO

What does it mean to reverse diabetes?

Reversing diabetes refers to the achievement of a state where blood sugar levels return to normal or near-normal levels, and the symptoms and complications associated with diabetes are significantly mitigated. While it's essential to clarify that Type 1 diabetes, characterised by the immune system attacking insulin-producing cells, cannot be reversed, the focus here is primarily on Type 2 diabetes.

Understanding Type 2 Diabetes:

Insulin Resistance: Type 2 diabetes often involves insulin resistance, where cells don't respond effectively to insulin, leading to elevated blood sugar levels.

Lifestyle Factors: Factors such as sedentary lifestyles, poor dietary choices, and obesity contribute to the development of Type 2 diabetes.

Reversal Strategies:

Healthy Eating:

Adopting a balanced, nutrient-dense diet with an emphasis on whole foods.

Managing portion sizes and choosing foods with a lower glycemic index.

Weight Management:

Insulin sensitivity can be enhanced by reaching and maintaining a healthy weight.

Regular physical activity supports weight management and enhances insulin function.

Regular Exercise:

Engaging in physical activity enhances insulin sensitivity and lowers blood sugar levels

Combining aerobic exercises with strength training provides comprehensive benefits.

Medication Management:

Under the guidance of healthcare professionals, medication adjustments or discontinuation might be possible as blood sugar levels improve.

Blood Sugar Monitoring:

Regular monitoring is crucial to track progress and adjust lifestyle or medication accordingly.

Stress Management:

Chronic stress can impact blood sugar levels; stress reduction techniques contribute to overall well-being.

Education and Support:

Understanding the condition and making informed lifestyle choices are vital for long-term success.

Support from healthcare professionals, diabetes educators, and peer groups enhances the journey.

Indicators of Reversal:

Normalised Blood Sugar Levels:

Fasting blood sugar and HbA1c levels within a normal or pre-diabetic range.

Improved Insulin Sensitivity:

Cells respond more effectively to insulin.

Symptom Relief:

Reduction or elimination of diabetes symptoms like excessive thirst, frequent urination, and fatigue.

Reduced Medication Dependency:

Gradual reduction or elimination of diabetes medications under medical supervision.

Importance of Sustaining Reversal:

Lifestyle Continuity:

Long-term success requires the continuation of healthy habits and regular monitoring.

Regular Check-ups:

Ongoing medical supervision ensures sustained well-being.

Preventing Relapse:

Avoiding lifestyle factors that contribute to diabetes relapse is crucial.

In conclusion, reversing diabetes in the context of Type 2 involves comprehensive lifestyle changes, focusing on nutrition, physical activity, and overall health. It's a dynamic process that requires commitment, education, and ongoing support to achieve and sustain positive outcomes. Always consult with healthcare professionals for personalised guidance and monitoring throughout this journey.

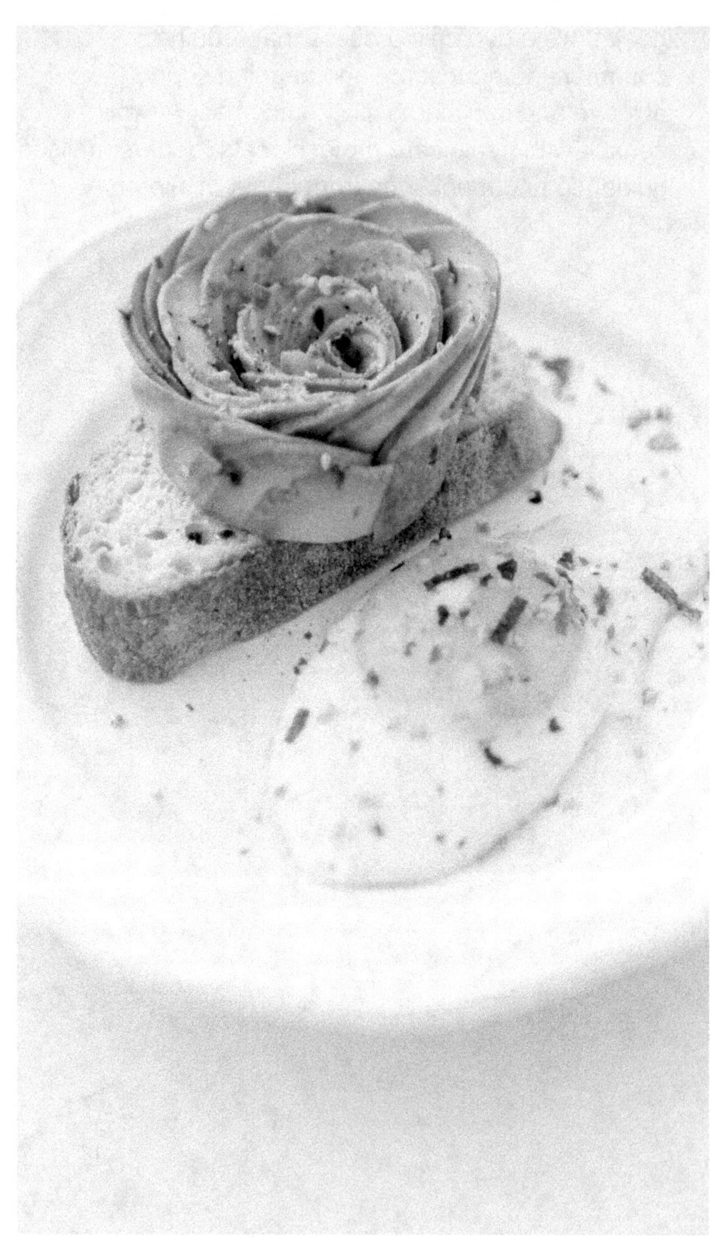

CHAPTER THREE

The Role of Nutrition in Reversing Diabetes

Nutrition plays a pivotal role in the reversal of diabetes, particularly in the context of Type 2 diabetes. A well-balanced and strategic approach to dietary choices can significantly impact blood sugar levels, insulin sensitivity, and overall metabolic health. Here's an exploration of the key aspects of nutrition in the reversal of diabetes:

1. Balancing Macronutrients:

Carbohydrates: Choosing complex carbohydrates with a low glycemic index helps regulate blood sugar. Emphasising whole grains, vegetables, and legumes is beneficial.

Proteins: Including lean protein sources supports satiety and muscle health without causing rapid spikes in blood sugar.

Fats: Prioritising healthy fats, such as those from avocados, nuts, and olive oil, contributes to overall heart health.

2. Portion Control:

Managing portion sizes helps regulate calorie intake and prevents overconsumption, aiding in weight management and blood sugar control.

3. Fibre-Rich Foods:

High-fibre foods like fruits, vegetables, and whole grains slow down the absorption of glucose, promoting stable blood sugar levels.

4. Reducing Added Sugars:

Minimising the intake of processed foods and beverages with added sugars helps prevent blood sugar spikes and supports overall health.

5. Strategic Meal Timing:

Distributing meals evenly throughout the day and avoiding prolonged periods without food can help regulate blood sugar levels.

6. Emphasis on Nutrient-Dense Foods:

Prioritising nutrient-dense foods ensures that the body receives essential vitamins and minerals for overall health.

7. Hydration:

Staying adequately hydrated is crucial for metabolic function. Water is the preferred beverage, while sugary drinks should be limited.

8. Moderating Alcohol Intake:

Consuming alcohol in moderation is advised, as excessive intake can affect blood sugar levels and overall health.

9. Customization to Individual Needs:

Recognizing that nutritional needs vary among individuals, personalised dietary plans are essential. Factors like age, activity level, and specific health conditions should be considered.

10. Continuous Monitoring and Adjustment:

Regularly monitoring blood sugar levels allows for adjustments in the diet as needed. This ensures that the nutritional approach aligns with individual health goals.

11. Nutritional Education:

Providing individuals with diabetes education about the impact of different foods on blood sugar levels empowers them to make informed choices and sustain a healthy lifestyle.

12. Collaboration with Healthcare Professionals:

Working closely with healthcare professionals, including dietitians and nutritionists, ensures that dietary plans are tailored to individual needs and are aligned with overall health goals.

In essence, nutrition serves as a cornerstone in the reversal of diabetes. A thoughtful and balanced approach to dietary choices, coupled with other lifestyle modifications, can contribute significantly to improved blood sugar control, enhanced insulin sensitivity, and overall well-being. It's essential for individuals to approach dietary changes as part of a comprehensive strategy, seeking guidance from healthcare professionals to achieve sustained and positive outcomes.

CHAPTER FOUR

Kitchen essentials and cooking techniques

Achieving diabetes reversal involves incorporating key ingredients into your diet that support blood sugar control, improve insulin sensitivity, and contribute to overall metabolic health. Here's an extensive exploration of these essential ingredients:

1. Whole Grains:

Examples: Quinoa, brown rice, oats

Role: Provide complex carbohydrates, fibre, and essential nutrients without causing rapid spikes in blood sugar.

2. Leafy Green Vegetables:

Examples: Spinach, kale, Swiss chard

Role: Rich in fibre, vitamins, and minerals; low in calories; and contribute to stable blood sugar levels.

3. Berries:

Examples: Blueberries, strawberries, raspberries

Role: Packed with antioxidants, fibre, and natural sweetness without causing significant blood sugar spikes.

4. Legumes:

Examples: Lentils, chickpeas, black beans

Role: Excellent sources of plant-based protein and fibre, promoting satiety and blood sugar control.

5. Nuts and Seeds:

Examples: Almonds, chia seeds, flaxseeds

Role: Provide healthy fats, protein, and fibre; contribute to a feeling of fullness and help regulate blood sugar.

6. Fatty Fish:

Examples: Salmon, mackerel, sardines

Role: Rich in omega-3 fatty acids, supporting heart health and potentially improving insulin sensitivity.

7. Lean Proteins:

Examples: Skinless poultry, tofu, lean cuts of meat

Role: Essential for muscle health, helps control hunger, and regulates blood sugar levels.

8. Non-Starchy Vegetables:

Examples: Broccoli, cauliflower, bell peppers

Role: Low in carbohydrates, high in fibre and nutrients, contribute to a balanced and low-glycemic diet.

9. Cinnamon:

Role: Some studies suggest that cinnamon may help improve insulin sensitivity and lower blood sugar levels.

10. Turmeric:

Role: Contains curcumin, which has anti-inflammatory properties and may contribute to improved insulin function.

11. Low-Fat Dairy or Dairy Alternatives:

Examples: Greek yoghourt, almond milk

Role: Source of calcium and protein without excessive saturated fats; supports overall metabolic health.

12. Avocado:

Role: Provides healthy monounsaturated fats, fiber, and various nutrients; supports heart health.

13. Garlic:

Role: Contains allicin, which may have beneficial effects on insulin sensitivity.

14. Green Tea:

Role: Rich in antioxidants, may help improve insulin sensitivity and reduce blood sugar levels.

15. Apple Cider Vinegar:

Role: Some studies suggest it may help lower fasting blood sugar levels and improve insulin sensitivity.

16. Probiotics:

Sources: Yogurt, kefir, fermented foods

Role: Support gut health, potentially influencing metabolic function and insulin sensitivity.

17. Water:

Role: Staying hydrated is crucial for overall health and helps maintain proper metabolic function.

18. Eggs:

Role: High-quality protein source, rich in nutrients, and may contribute to satiety.

19. Mushrooms:

Role: Low in carbohydrates, rich in vitamins and minerals, and may have anti-inflammatory properties.

20. Sweet Potatoes:

Role: A nutrient-dense, low-glycemic carbohydrate source, providing fibre, vitamins, and minerals.

Considerations:

Individualization: Dietary needs vary, and it's crucial to tailor the diet to individual preferences, health status, and cultural considerations.

Balanced Approach: Combining these ingredients in a balanced manner supports an overall healthy and sustainable dietary pattern.

Incorporating these key ingredients into a well-rounded and balanced diet, along with regular physical activity, can contribute significantly to the reversal and management of diabetes. It's advisable

to consult with healthcare professionals or a
registered dietitian to create a personalised nutrition
plan tailored to individual health goals and needs.

Designing a kitchen for individuals focusing on the
reversal of diabetes involves thoughtful consideration
of essential tools and cooking techniques that
promote healthy, flavorful meals. Here's an
exploration of key kitchen essentials and cooking
techniques tailored for a diabetes reversal approach.

CHAPTER FIVE

Kitchen Essential

Quality Cookware:

Invest in non-stick pans, stainless steel pots, and oven-safe bakeware for cooking versatility with minimal added fats.

Sharp Knives:

Precise knife work ensures efficient preparation of fresh vegetables and lean proteins.

Food Processor or Blender:

These appliances facilitate the creation of nutrient-rich sauces, dips, and smoothies without added sugars or unhealthy fats.

Measuring Tools:

Accurate measuring cups and spoons help maintain portion control and monitor ingredient quantities.

Cutting Boards:

Differentiate cutting boards for various food groups to prevent cross-contamination.

Storage Containers:

Use a variety of containers for portioning meals, storing leftovers, and organising prepped ingredients.

Slow Cooker or Instant Pot:

These devices simplify cooking while preserving flavours and nutrients, making meal preparation efficient.

Digital Kitchen Scale:

Useful for precise measurement of ingredients, especially when managing carbohydrates.

Herbs and Spices:

A well-stocked spice rack enhances flavour without relying on added salt or sugar.

Steamer Basket:

Ideal for retaining the nutritional value and crisp texture of vegetables through gentle steaming.

Cooking Techniques:

Grilling and Broiling:

Enhance flavours without excess fats by grilling or broiling lean proteins and vegetables.

Roasting and Baking:

Roast vegetables and bake lean proteins for depth of flavour without unnecessary added oils.

Stir-Frying:

Quick and nutritious, stir-frying uses minimal oil and high heat for preserving the texture and nutrients of ingredients.

Steaming:

Retain nutrients and natural flavours by steaming vegetables, fish, and whole grains.

Sauteing:

Lightly sautéing ingredients in heart-healthy oils can build layers of flavour in dishes.

Poaching:

A gentle cooking method using simmering liquid like water or broth, preserving tenderness and moisture in proteins.

Blending and Pureeing:

Create smooth textures for sauces, soups, and smoothies with whole, fresh ingredients.

Marinating:

Infuse flavour into proteins using marinades with herbs, spices, and vinegar, reducing the need for added sugars or salts.

Portion Control:

Maintain awareness of portion sizes to support blood sugar regulation and overall health.

Incorporating Fresh Ingredients:

Prioritise whole, fresh foods to maximise nutritional value and minimise processed additives.

Considerations:

Adaptability: Recipes and techniques should be adaptable to individual preferences, dietary restrictions, and cultural backgrounds.

Education: Provide cooking tips and nutritional insights to empower individuals in making informed, health-conscious choices.

Creating a kitchen environment tailored for diabetes reversal involves a combination of practical tools and mindful cooking techniques. By incorporating these essentials, individuals can embark on a flavorful and nutritious culinary journey that supports their health goals.

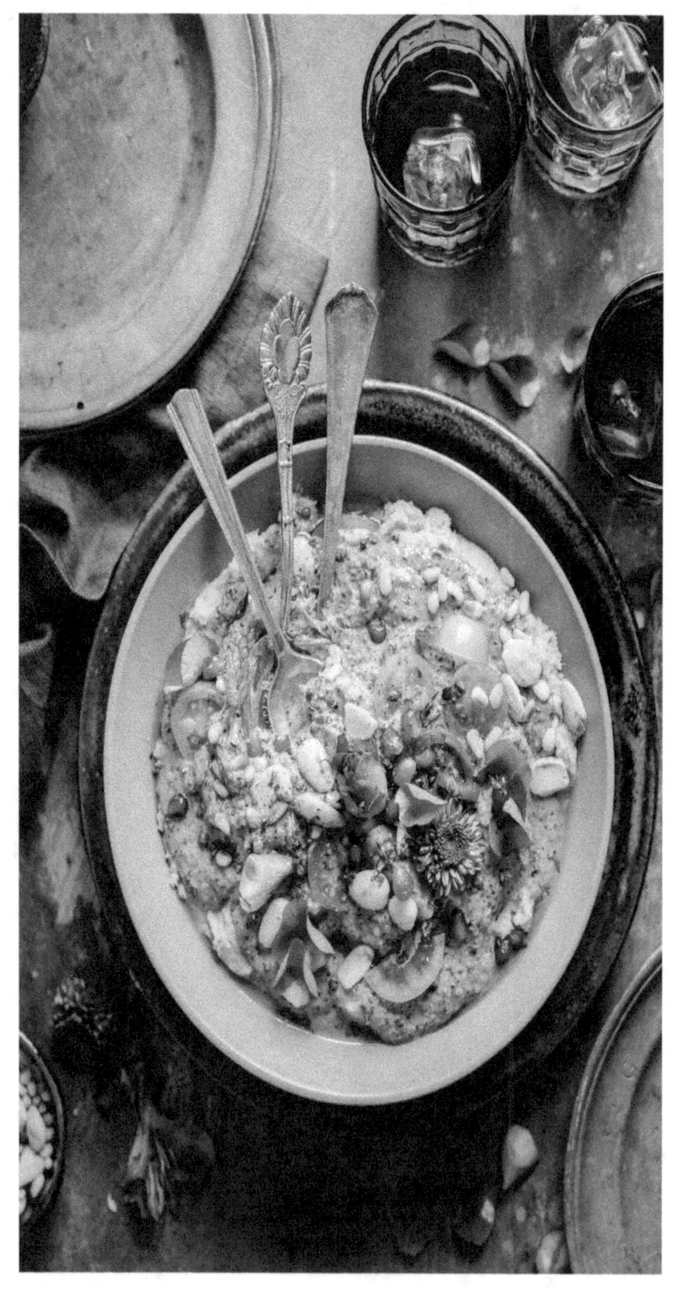

CHAPTER SIX

Recipes for breakfasts that heals

Certainly! It's important to note that managing diabetes involves a holistic approach, including a balanced diet and regular exercise. Here are two breakfast recipes that incorporate nutrient-dense ingredients:

Quinoa Breakfast Bowl:

Ingredients: Quinoa, eggs, spinach, cherry tomatoes, avocado.

Instructions: Cook quinoa according to package instructions. Sauté spinach and cherry tomatoes, then mix with cooked quinoa. Top with poached or fried eggs and sliced avocado. Quinoa provides complex carbs and fibre, supporting stable blood sugar levels.

Greek Yoghurt Parfait:

Ingredients: Greek yoghurt, mixed berries, almonds, flaxseeds.

Instructions: Layer Greek yoghurt with mixed berries, chopped almonds, and a sprinkle of flaxseeds. Greek yoghurt is rich in protein, and the berries provide antioxidants. Almonds and flax seeds add healthy fats and fibre, contributing to blood sugar control.

Always get the advice of a medical expert before making any dietary changes.

Always get the advice of a medical expert before making any dietary changes.

CHAPTER SEVEN

Recipes for lunches for wellness

Certainly! Here are two lunch recipes that focus on nutrient-dense, diabetes-friendly ingredients:

Salmon and Quinoa Salad:

Ingredients: Grilled salmon, cooked quinoa, mixed greens, cherry tomatoes, cucumber, feta cheese.

Instructions: Combine grilled salmon with quinoa, mixed greens, sliced cherry tomatoes, cucumber, and crumbled feta cheese. Drizzle with olive oil and lemon juice. This dish provides protein, healthy fats, and fibre.

Vegetable Stir-Fry with Tofu:

Ingredients: Tofu, broccoli, bell peppers, carrots, snap peas, garlic, ginger.

Instructions: Stir-fry tofu with a mix of broccoli, bell peppers, carrots, snap peas, garlic, and ginger. Season with low-sodium soy sauce or a light vinaigrette. Tofu adds protein, and the colourful vegetables provide vitamins and fibre.

Remember to tailor these recipes to individual dietary needs, and it's essential to consult with a healthcare professional for personalised advice on managing diabetes.

CHAPTER EIGHT

Nourishing soup recipes

Certainly! Soups can be nourishing and satisfying while also being low in carbohydrates and high in nutrients, making them suitable for diabetes management. Here are two nourishing soup recipes:

Vegetable and Lentil Soup:

Ingredients:

1 cup green or brown lentils, rinsed

1 onion, diced

2 carrots, diced

2 celery stalks, diced

2 cloves garlic, minced

6 cups vegetable broth

1 can diced tomatoes (low-sodium)

2 teaspoons dried thyme

1 teaspoon ground cumin

Salt and pepper to taste

Olive oil for sautéing

Instructions:

Heat the olive oil in a big pot to a medium temperature. Add diced onions, carrots, celery, and garlic. Sauté until softened, about 5-7 minutes.

Add lentils, vegetable broth, diced tomatoes, thyme, and cumin to the pot. Bring to a boil, then reduce heat and simmer for about 25-30 minutes, or until lentils are tender.

Season with salt and pepper to taste. Adjust seasoning if necessary.

Serve hot and garnish with fresh herbs if desired. This soup is rich in fibre, protein, and vitamins, making it a great option for stabilising blood sugar levels.

Chicken and Vegetable Soup:

Ingredients:

1 lb boneless, skinless chicken breasts or thighs, diced

1 onion, diced

2 carrots, diced

2 celery stalks, diced

2 cloves garlic, minced

6 cups chicken broth (low-sodium)

1 cup diced tomatoes (low-sodium)

1 teaspoon dried thyme

1 teaspoon dried rosemary

Salt and pepper to taste

Olive oil for sautéing

Instructions:

Olive oil should be heated over medium heat in a big pot. Add diced onions, carrots, celery, and garlic. Sauté until softened, about 5-7 minutes.

Cook the chopped chicken in the pot until it turns brown on all sides.

Pour in chicken broth and diced tomatoes. Add dried thyme and rosemary. Bring to a boil, then reduce heat and simmer for about 20-25 minutes, or until chicken is cooked through.

Season with salt and pepper to taste. Adjust seasoning if necessary.

Serve hot and garnish with fresh parsley if desired. This soup is protein-rich and packed with vegetables, making it a nutritious choice for individuals managing diabetes.

These soup recipes are versatile and can be customised with your favourite herbs, spices, and vegetables. Enjoy them as a comforting and nourishing meal option while supporting diabetes management.

CHAPTER NINE

Wholesome dinner recipes that restore

Here's a wholesome dinner recipe that focuses on nutrient-dense ingredients and is suitable for managing diabetes:

Baked Salmon with Roasted Vegetables:

Ingredients:

4 salmon fillets

2 tablespoons olive oil

2 cloves garlic, minced

1 teaspoon lemon zest

1 tablespoon lemon juice

Salt and pepper to taste

4 cups mixed vegetables (such as broccoli, bell peppers, zucchini, and cherry tomatoes)

1 tablespoon balsamic vinegar

Fresh herbs for garnish (optional)

Instructions:

Preheat the oven to 400°F (200°C).

Combine the olive oil, minced garlic, lemon zest, and lemon juice in a small bowl. Season the salmon fillets with salt and pepper, then brush them with the olive oil mixture.

Arrange the salmon fillets onto a parchment paper-lined baking sheet. Bake the salmon for 12 to 15 minutes, or until it is cooked through and flake readily with a fork, in an oven that has been warmed.

As the salmon bakes, get the roasted vegetables ready. Combine salt, pepper, olive oil, and balsamic vinegar with the mixed vegetables. Spread them out on a separate baking sheet.

Roast the vegetables in the oven for 20-25 minutes, or until they are tender and lightly browned, stirring halfway through.

Once the salmon and vegetables are done, serve them hot, garnished with fresh herbs if desired.

This dinner recipe provides a balanced combination of protein, healthy fats, and fibre-rich vegetables. Salmon is rich in omega-3 fatty acids, which have been shown to have beneficial effects on heart health and may help improve insulin sensitivity. The roasted vegetables offer an array of vitamins, minerals, and antioxidants while keeping the meal low in carbohydrates.

As always, it's important to consult with a healthcare professional for personalised dietary recommendations and to monitor blood sugar levels while managing diabetes. Enjoy this delicious and nutritious dinner option!

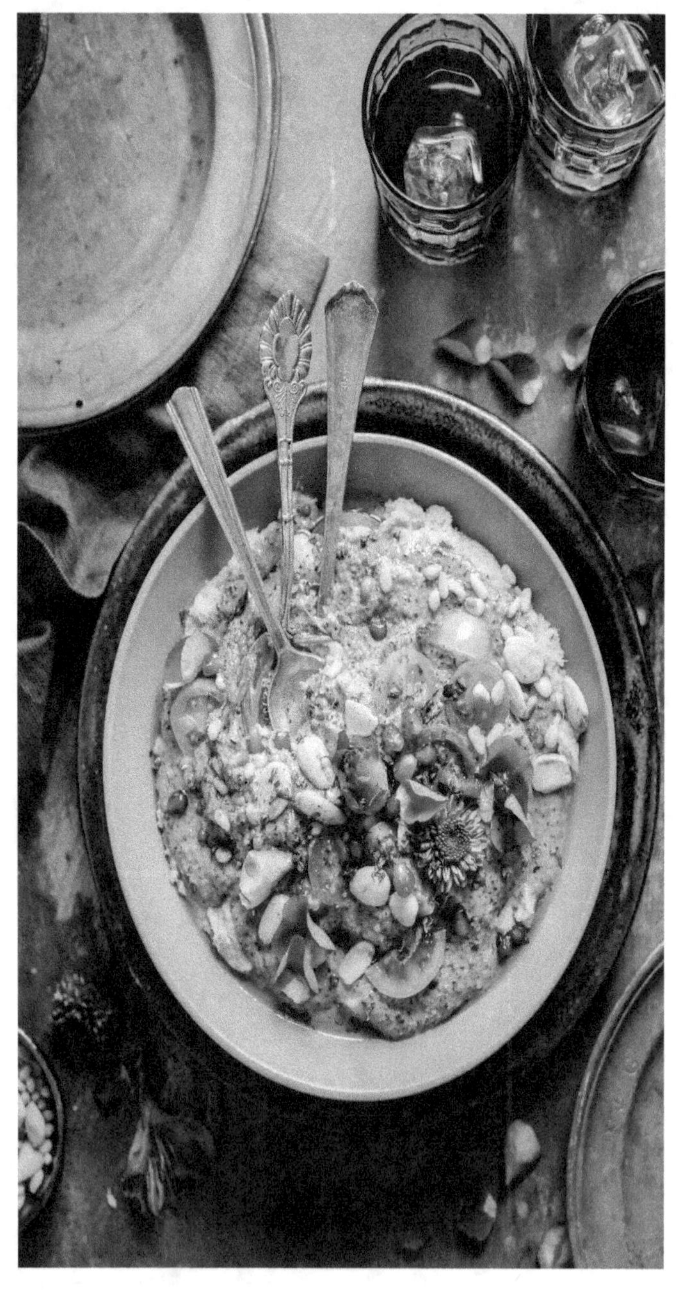

CHAPTER TEN

Satisfying vegetarian options

Here's a wholesome vegetarian recipe that's suitable for managing diabetes:

Quinoa Stuffed Bell Peppers:

Ingredients:

4 large bell peppers, any colour

1 cup quinoa, rinsed

2 cups vegetable broth

One can (15 oz) of rinsed and drained black beans

1 cup corn kernels (fresh or frozen)

1 onion, diced

2 cloves garlic, minced

1 teaspoon ground cumin

1 teaspoon chilli powder

1/2 teaspoon paprika

Salt and pepper to taste

1 cup shredded cheese (optional, choose low-fat or vegan cheese for a healthier option)

Fresh cilantro or parsley for garnish (optional)

Olive oil for cooking

Instructions:

Preheat the oven to 375°F (190°C). Grease a baking dish with olive oil.

Slice off the bell peppers' tops, then take out the seeds and membranes. Cut-side up, put the peppers in the baking dish that has been prepared.

Quinoa and vegetable broth should be combined in a medium saucepan. Bring to a boil, then reduce heat, cover, and simmer for about 15 minutes, or until the quinoa is cooked and the liquid is absorbed.

In a big skillet over medium heat, warm the olive oil. Add the chopped onion and simmer for about 5 minutes, or until transparent. One minute after adding the minced garlic, continue to sauté.

Add cooked quinoa, black beans, corn kernels, ground cumin, chilli powder, paprika, salt, and pepper to the skillet. Cook for a few more minutes, stirring to mix well, until well cooked.

Stuff the quinoa mixture into the hollowed-out bell peppers, pressing down gently to pack the filling.

If using cheese, sprinkle it over the stuffed bell peppers.

Once the oven is preheated, bake the baking dish covered with foil for 25 to 30 minutes, or until the peppers are soft.

Remove the foil and bake for an additional 5-10 minutes to melt the cheese and allow the tops of the peppers to brown slightly.

Before serving, take out of the oven and allow it to cool for a few minutes. Garnish with fresh cilantro or parsley if desired.

These quinoa stuffed bell peppers are rich in fibre, protein, vitamins, and minerals, making them a nutritious and satisfying meal for individuals managing diabetes. Enjoy this wholesome vegetarian dish as part of a balanced diet.

CHAPTER ELEVEN

Balanced snacks and side dishes recipes

Certainly! Here are two wholesome and balanced recipes, one for a snack and one for a side dish, suitable for managing diabetes:

Snack: Hummus and Veggie Platter

Ingredients:

1 cup hummus (choose a variety with minimal added sugars)

Baby carrots

Cherry tomatoes

Cucumber slices

Bell pepper strips (assorted colours)

Whole grain crackers

Instructions:

Arrange baby carrots, cherry tomatoes, cucumber slices, bell pepper strips, and whole grain crackers on a platter.

Present beside a hummus bowl for dipping.

This snack is rich in fibre, healthy fats, and a variety of vitamins and minerals. The combination of vegetables and hummus provides a satisfying and blood sugar-friendly option.

Side Dish: Roasted Sweet Potato Wedges

Ingredients:

2 large sweet potatoes, washed and cut into wedges

2 tablespoons olive oil

1 teaspoon smoked paprika

1 teaspoon garlic powder

1/2 teaspoon cinnamon

Salt and pepper to taste

Instructions:

Preheat the oven to 400°F (200°C).

In a large bowl, toss sweet potato wedges with olive oil, smoked paprika, garlic powder, cinnamon, salt, and pepper until evenly coated.

Arrange the sweet potato wedges on a baking sheet that has been lined with parchment paper in a single layer.

Roast in the preheated oven for 25-30 minutes or until the wedges are golden brown and tender, flipping halfway through.

Remove from the oven and serve hot.

These roasted sweet potato wedges are a great side dish option. Sweet potatoes provide complex carbohydrates, fibre , and essential nutrients, making them a nutritious choice for individuals managing diabetes. The combination of spices adds flavour without the need for excessive added sugars or salt.

CHAPTER NINE

Recipes for Decadent yet diabetes friendly desserts

Creating decadent yet diabetes-friendly desserts involves focusing on whole, nutrient-dense ingredients and mindful portion control. Here's a recipe for a delicious and diabetes-friendly dessert:

Dark Chocolate Avocado Mousse:

Ingredients:

2 ripe avocados

1/4 cup unsweetened cocoa powder

1/4 cup dark chocolate chips (70% cocoa or higher)

1/4 cup almond milk (unsweetened)

2-3 tablespoons pure maple syrup or a sugar substitute of your choice

1 teaspoon vanilla extract

Pinch of salt

Fresh berries for garnish (optional)

Instructions:

Melt the dark chocolate chips using a double boiler or in short intervals in the microwave, stirring until smooth.

In a blender or food processor, combine the ripe avocados, melted chocolate, cocoa powder, almond milk, maple syrup (or sugar substitute), vanilla extract, and a pinch of salt.

Blend until the mixture is creamy and well combined. You may need to stop and scrape down the sides of the blender or food processor to ensure all ingredients are incorporated.

Taste the mousse and adjust sweetness if necessary by adding more maple syrup or sugar substitute.

Once the mixture is smooth, spoon it into serving glasses or bowls.

Chill in the refrigerator for at least 1-2 hours or until set.

Before serving, garnish with fresh berries if desired.

This dark chocolate avocado mousse is rich in healthy fats from avocados and antioxidants from dark chocolate. The use of natural sweeteners and a moderate portion size makes it a diabetes-friendly dessert option.

Remember to enjoy desserts in moderation and consult with a healthcare professional for personalised advice on managing diabetes.

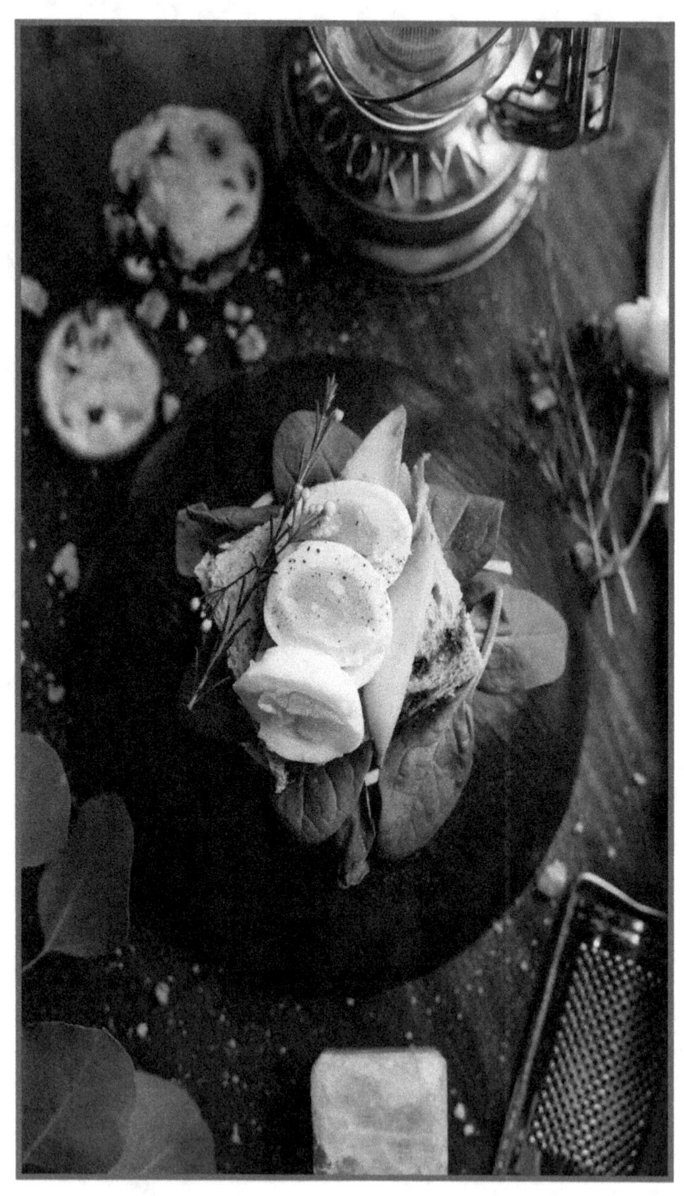

CHAPTER TEN

Fruits-based delicacies for sweet cravings

Certainly! Here are two sumptuous recipes for fruit-based delicacies that can be enjoyed as part of a diabetes-friendly diet:

1. Berry and Yogurt Parfait:

Ingredients:

1 cup Greek yoghourt (unsweetened)

1 cup mixed berries (strawberries, blueberries, raspberries)

1 tablespoon chia seeds

1 tablespoon chopped nuts (almonds, walnuts)

1 teaspoon honey or a sugar substitute

Fresh mint leaves for garnish (optional)

Instructions:

Greek yoghurt should be layered at the bottom of a glass or bowl.

Cover the yoghurt with a layer of mixed berries.

Sprinkle chia seeds and chopped nuts over the berries.

Drizzle honey or a sugar substitute over the layers.

Continue layering until the entire glass or bowl is filled.

Garnish with fresh mint leaves if desired.

When ready to eat, serve straight away or store in the refrigerator.

2. Grilled Pineapple with Cinnamon:

Ingredients:

One pineapple, cored, peeled, and sliced into rings

1 tablespoon coconut oil (melted)

1 teaspoon ground cinnamon

Fresh lime wedges for serving

Instructions:

Set a grill pan or grill at a medium heat.

Brush pineapple rings with melted coconut oil.

Grill the pineapple rings for 2-3 minutes per side or until they have grill marks and are slightly caramelised.

Remove from the grill and sprinkle ground cinnamon over the grilled pineapple.

Serve warm with fresh lime wedges on the side.

Both recipes incorporate fruits that are rich in fibre, vitamins, and antioxidants, which can be beneficial for individuals managing diabetes. The use of natural sweeteners and healthy fats makes these delicacies a tasty and diabetes-friendly treat. As always, it's important to consider individual dietary needs and consult with a healthcare professional for personalised advice.

CHAPTER ELEVEN

Weekly meals plans for diabetes reversal

Creating a well-balanced weekly meal plan for managing diabetes involves incorporating a variety of nutrient-dense foods. Here's a sample plan:

Day 1:

Breakfast: Vegetable Omelette (Eggs, spinach, tomatoes, bell peppers)

Lunch: Quinoa Salad with Grilled Chicken (Quinoa, mixed greens, cherry tomatoes, cucumber)

Snack: Greek Yoghourt

 with Berries

Dinner: Baked Salmon with Roasted Vegetables (Salmon, broccoli, carrots, bell peppers)

Day 2:

Breakfast: Chia Seed Pudding (Chia seeds, almond milk, berries)

Lunch: Lentil Soup with Whole Grain Roll

Snack: Hummus with Veggie Sticks

Dinner: Stir-Fried Tofu with Vegetables (Tofu, broccoli, bell peppers, snap peas)

Day 3:

Breakfast: Banana and Almond Butter Overnight Oats

Lunch: Chickpea Salad (Chickpeas, cherry tomatoes, cucumber, feta cheese)

Snack: Nuts and Seeds Mix

Dinner: Quinoa Stuffed Bell Peppers (Quinoa, black beans, corn, bell peppers)

Day 4:

Breakfast: Whole Grain Toast with Avocado and
Poached Egg

Lunch: Vegetable and Lentil Soup with Whole Grain
Crackers

Snack: Cottage Cheese with Pineapple

Dinner: steamed asparagus and grilled chicken with
sweet potato wedges.

Day 5:

Breakfast: Smoothie Bowl (Spinach, banana, berries,
almond milk)

Lunch: Brown Rice Bowl with Black Beans, Salsa,
and Avocado

Snack: Apple Slices with Almond Butter

Dinner: Baked Cod with Quinoa Pilaf and Roasted
Brussels Sprouts

Day 6:

Breakfast: Yoghurt Parfait with Mixed Berries, Chia Seeds, and Granola

Lunch: Spinach and Feta Stuffed Chicken Breast with Steamed Broccoli

Snack: Carrot Sticks with Hummus

Supper: brown rice and chickpea curry with aubergine.

Day 7:

Breakfast: Buckwheat Pancakes with Fresh Fruit Topping

Lunch: Turkey and Vegetable Lettuce Wraps

Snack: Greek Yoghurt with Walnuts and a Drizzle of Honey

Dinner: Lentil and Vegetable Stir-Fry with Cauliflower Rice

Remember to adjust portion sizes based on individual dietary needs and consult with a healthcare professional for personalised advice on managing diabetes. Additionally, regular physical activity is an important component of diabetes management, so incorporating exercise into your routine is encouraged.

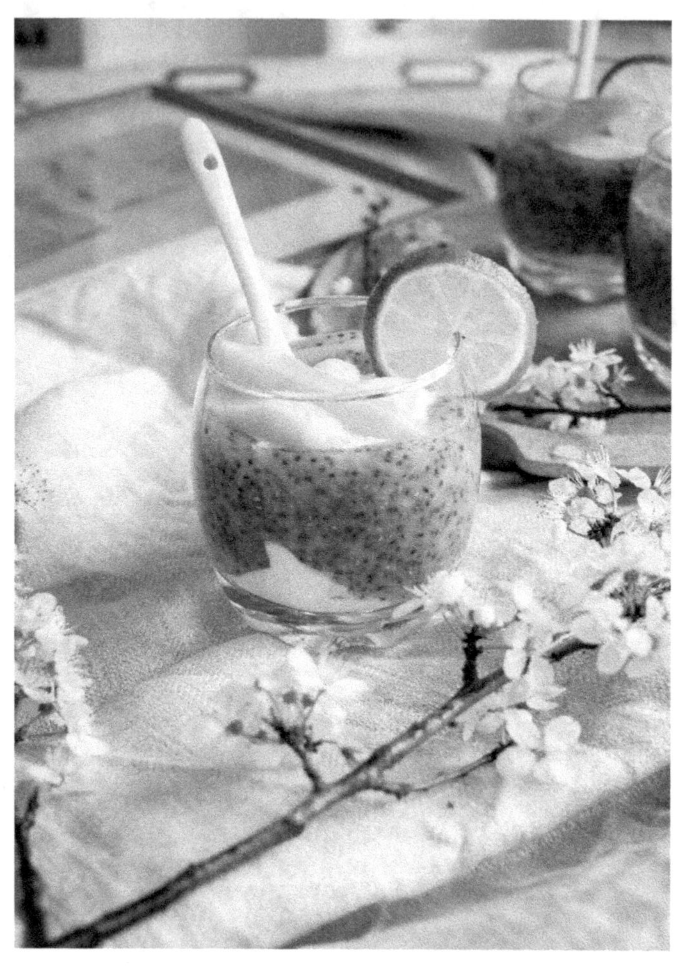

CHAPTER TWELVE

Tips for dining out on social occasions

Dining out on social occasions while managing diabetes requires thoughtful choices to maintain blood sugar levels. Here are extensive tips to navigate such situations:

1. Plan Ahead:

Try to look over the menu online before visiting the restaurant.

Consider calling the restaurant in advance to inquire about healthy options or any modifications that can be made to accommodate your dietary needs.

2. Choose Wisely:

Lean protein sources such as fish, grilled chicken, or lean meat cuts should be preferred.

Select whole grains, such as brown rice or quinoa, over refined carbohydrates.

Load up on non-starchy vegetables, salads, and steamed options.

3. Be Mindful of Portions:

In order to avoid overeating, request a to-go box at the start of the dinner and set aside some food to take home.

4. Control Your Carbs:

Be cautious with bread and appetisers. Consider skipping them or having a small portion.

Choose complex carbohydrates and monitor portion sizes to control your carbohydrate intake.

5. Monitor Sauces and Dressings:

Ask for sauces and dressings on the side, allowing you to control the amount you consume.

Opt for vinaigrettes or tomato-based sauces instead of creamy or sugary options.

6. Hydrate Smartly:

Choose water, unsweetened tea, or other non-caloric beverages to stay hydrated.

Limit sugary drinks, as they can quickly raise blood sugar levels.

7. Mindful Eating:

Eat slowly and savour each bite. This can help you recognize when you're satisfied, preventing overeating.

Put your fork down between bites to avoid rushing through the meal.

8. Dessert Decisions:

Share desserts with others to enjoy a taste without consuming a full portion.

Consider fresh fruit or a small serving of a diabetes-friendly dessert if available.

9. Stay Active:

If possible, suggest activities that involve movement after the meal, such as a short walk.

Physical activity can help regulate blood sugar levels and aid digestion.

10. Communicate with Others:

Inform your dining companions about your dietary preferences and the importance of making healthy choices.

Choose restaurants that offer a variety of options, making it easier for everyone to find something they enjoy.

11. Monitor Alcohol Intake:

If consuming alcohol, do so in moderation. Consider lower-carb options like dry wine or spirits with sugar-free mixers.

Always monitor blood sugar levels closely when drinking alcohol.

12. Don't Be Afraid to Ask:

Don't hesitate to ask the server about ingredients or how dishes are prepared.

Most restaurants are accommodating to dietary requests, and it's crucial to prioritise your health.

By being proactive and making thoughtful choices, you can enjoy social occasions while managing diabetes effectively. Always listen to your body, monitor blood sugar levels regularly, and consult with healthcare professionals for personalised advice.

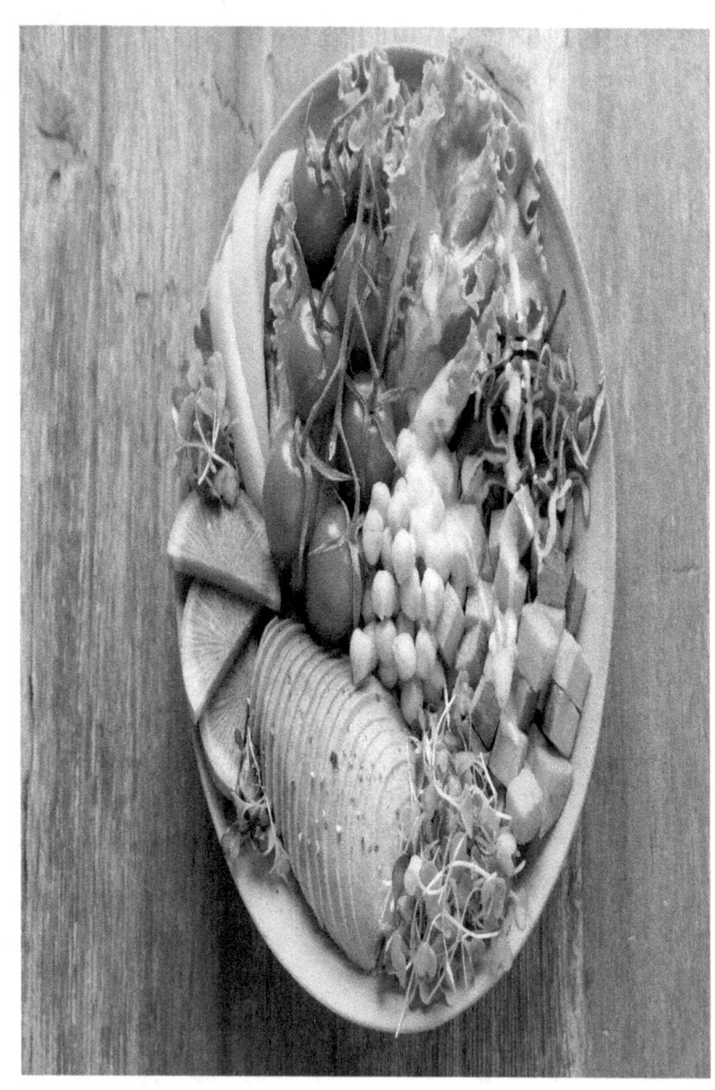

CHAPTER THIRTEEN

Conclusion

In conclusion, the journey towards reversing diabetes is a multifaceted endeavour that intertwines dietary choices, lifestyle modifications, and a commitment to overall well-being. Embracing a balanced and nutrient-dense diet, rich in whole foods and mindful of carbohydrates, lays a robust foundation. Coupled with regular physical activity, stress management, and adequate sleep, this holistic approach becomes a powerful catalyst for diabetes reversal.

It is essential to foster a partnership with healthcare professionals, creating a collaborative and informed strategy tailored to individual needs. Regular monitoring of blood sugar levels, coupled with adjustments in response to the body's signals, empowers individuals to make informed decisions on their path to wellness.

Reversing diabetes is not a linear journey but rather a continuous commitment to self-care. Celebrating victories, no matter how small, and learning from challenges contribute to a sustainable and resilient approach. As the journey unfolds, it is crucial to acknowledge the profound impact of lifestyle choices on health and the empowerment that comes from taking charge of one's well-being.

In the pursuit of diabetes reversal, remember that each step towards a healthier lifestyle is a stride towards a brighter, more vibrant future. The resilience of the human body, coupled with mindful choices, creates a narrative of hope and transformation. Let this journey be a testament to the remarkable capacity of the human spirit to overcome and thrive, embracing a life of vitality, balance, and renewed well-being.